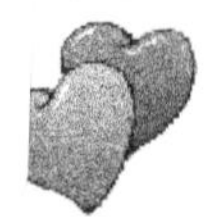

How To Find God's Will

Frances Hunter

Books By Charles and Frances Hunter

A Confession A Day Keeps The Devil Away
The Angel Book
Are You Tired?
Born Again! What Do You Mean?
Come Alive
Don't Be Afraid Of Fear
Follow Me
Go, Man, Go!
God's Answer To Fat...LOØSE IT!
God's Big "IF"
Handbook For Healing
Hang Loose With Jesus
Heart To Heart Flip Chart
Hot Line To Heaven
How To Find God's Will
How Do You Treat My Son Jesus?
How To Heal The Sick
How To Make Your Marriage Exciting
How To Pick A Perfect Husband...Or Wife
How To Receive And Maintain A Healing
How To Receive And Minister The Baptism With The Holy Spirit
If Charles And Frances Can Do It, YOU Can Do It, Too!
If You Really Love Me...
Impossible Miracles
Let This Mind Be In You
Memorizing Made Easy
Strength For Today
Supernatural Horizons
There Are Two Kinds Of...
The Two Sides Of A Coin
Why Should "I" Speak In Tongues?

ISBN 0-917726-58-8

Scripture quotations are taken from:
New King James Version (NKJV) ©1979, 1980, 1982 by Thomas Nelson, Inc., Nashville, TN.
The Living Bible, Paraphrased (TLB), ©1971 by Tyndale House Publishers, Wheaton, IL
The Authorized King James Version (KJV)
The Amplified Bible (Amp.), ©1954, 1958 by The Lockman Foundation

How To Find God's Will

Is there really a way to find God's will for your life so you don't have to grope and fumble around, learning by trial and error?

Does God want you to flub, botch and bungle His will and plan for your life?

No!

Does God want you to be miserable?

NO!

Does God make His will and plan for your life easy?

YES!

How do you find God's will?

God's will is His word! I heard that said a long time ago but didn't understand it then, so let me explain how I found out what it really means.

I met Jesus in a very small, rundown church but I thought it was the most beautiful church in the world after I saw it filled with the Person and Presence of God!

When Jesus came into my heart, two things came into my heart with Him: a hunger for the word of God which has never been satisfied, and a desire to be with Christians. I didn't want to read anything except God's word and I didn't want to talk to anyone who didn't want to hear about Jesus. My heart was hungry to glean everything I could from being with Christians. I went to everything that even remotely sounded like the name God or Jesus might be mentioned!

One time I went to a wedding, even though

I didn't really know the people involved. The church was so small that the pastor was also the janitor, the maid, the gardener and the secretary. He dispensed these jobs to anyone who would take them!

Since the wedding was on a Saturday night, the church needed to be swept for Sunday morning. Since I was right there, the pastor handed me a broom and asked me to sweep the church.

That was the first thing God ever told me to do! Sweep out a church! And a junky church, at that! Certainly a far cry from what anyone would anticipate who knew they had heard God place a call on their life!

When I was saved, I had a full-time, live-in maid who took care of all the household needs. She even met me at the front door after work and handed me a lighted cigarette and a martini. That changed very quickly! But here was a pastor asking me to sweep the floor like a hired hand! I didn't hesitate one minute, even though I honestly didn't know how to sweep. I looked at the broom like it was a monster but tackled it with all the energy I had. Someone told me later they laughed because I was trying to sweep left-handed and didn't get very far. Finally, in desperation, I started picking up the rice with my fingers because I didn't make much progress with the broom.

Many times we miss the will of God because we think the job He gives us is too menial. We visualize ourselves in flowing chiffon dresses on a pedestal high above hundreds of thousands of people clamoring to hear just one word drip from our honey lips. We see people fighting to just touch us because so much of God emanates from our body that they know just one finger on us will answer all their problems. We're so busy living in a dream world that we can't feel the broomstick that God is hitting us with right across the back of our legs!

God is saying, "Hey, look at this little task I've got for you! I can't trust you with the big ones until you take care of this little thing!" Still we go on dreaming, wondering why we can't find God's will for our lives!

We need to look right in front of our noses if we want to see the wonder and glory of God, instead of looking through a telescope down the road a million miles away!

Do you know what you need to put in front of your nose so you'll know what God wants you to do? The Word – the Bible – the scriptures! God's will for you is all wrapped up right there!

"Go into all the world and preach the gospel to *every creature"* (Mark 16:15) was one of the first scriptures I memorized. I didn't memorize the rest of it because then I didn't like that business about speaking in tongues, but I did like the part about sharing the gospel with every creature. I quickly discovered that leading people to Jesus was God's will for my life.

I started with my family. After I shared with them, I shared with friends. I was happy, because I was doing God's will for my life!

When I finished with my friends (and my

success wasn't too great just in case you're interested), I was happy because I was doing the will of God just exactly as His word said.

The hardest thing in the world is to witness to your family and friends, especially when you become a fanatic from the word "go" because they all knew you "when" and they all think it's a temporary thing that will wear off – at least that's what my family and friends thought... but I KEPT ON!

I looked around for the next thing God wanted me to do. He said, "Share with the people in the shopping center where your office is located!"

The last thing in the world I wanted to do was to share with my business associates who had already begun to look at me as though I had gone senile, but God's word said to share it with the whole world, so I started there. I lost a lot of customers but God always brought me lots more who were interested in hearing what I had to say about what Jesus could do in their lives!

We get bogged down in doing God's will for our lives simply because if we get rebuffed we often get discouraged and think we must be out of the will of God, when in reality God is just giving us a little "toughening-up" period!

God enlarged the circle of my activities after I shared with my business associates and I began witnessing in the community of Kendall, Florida, where I lived. Each night I picked out three calls to make, left my office at seven and returned around nine to complete the day's work in my printing company.

I thought that was God's will for my life and would be for the rest of my days, but because I was obedient to God, He once again enlarged the circle of my responsibility. I began teaching others how to lead people to Jesus!

I didn't realize at the time that God was increasing my sphere of activities from that first one-to-one basis to a larger ministry. *"...you have been faithful over a few things, I will make you ruler over many things."* (Matt. 25:23). Faithfulness in the little things opened my ministry to larger things.

As soon as I had taught others how to lead people to Jesus on a one-to-one basis, I began receiving invitations from churches in Miami. I thought the entire city of Miami was my ministry for the rest of my life. I knew I would never be able to complete that huge job but I was happy because I was doing what God had called me to do.

The next thing God gave me was invitations to churches throughout the state of Florida. That grew to invitations from churches in other states in the nation. It was on one of these trips that I met Charles, who was a part of God's plan, God's will, for my life.

After our marriage, God gave us the entire United States, and on the tenth anniversary of my salvation, I found myself standing in Manila Bay baptizing Filipinos. God had given us the whole world!

As the tears started streaming down my face

with the joy of the Lord because of the realization of what God had done in my life, I looked at Charles and said, "I wonder what would have happened if I hadn't done that first little thing God told me to do – sweep out the church!"

Charles simply said, "Nothing!"

And that's right!

God will never move you on in His will until you do the little menial task He has sitting right in front of you! He can't trust you to share with thousands until He can trust you to share with just one!

Disobedience to God's will can bring real disaster! Adam discovered that! God created Adam in His own image so that He could have fellowship with him!

God brought every beast of the field and every fowl of the air to Adam *"to see what he would call them. And whatever Adam called each living creature, that was its name"* (Genesis 2:19).

Adam was happy because he was doing God's will. He didn't have to plow the field, he didn't have to plant, he didn't have to gather, he didn't have to harvest, he didn't have to work, he didn't have to struggle or strain. He just stayed in the beautiful garden of Eden, enjoying all of God's abundance, all of God's prosperity and divine health! Everything that God had was given to Adam in perfection.

Then God said to him, *"Of every tree of the garden you may freely eat; but of the tree of the knowledge of good and evil you shall not eat, for in that day that you eat of it you shall surely die"* (Gen. 2:16,17).

Then God said it wasn't good for man to live alone, so he created a woman from Adam's rib. Then God had two people in His perfect will. They were obedient to Him, to His purpose, to His laws and to His thinking.

They walked and talked with God! They were abundantly happy and so was God. There was nothing to be afraid of because they were walking in the will of God and there is no fear in the will of God. There was no reason for them to ever have anything except the joy of the Lord, but...

The one who comes to steal, to kill and to destroy sneaked into the beautiful Garden of Eden and he's still sneaking around today! The minute the devil sees everything going according to the will of God, he comes slinking in, not in the shape of a serpent, but in one form or another, trying to tempt us from doing the will of God.

Adam and Eve had everything going for them, and so do we, until we listen to the temptations of the devil!

God told Adam and Eve in very simple terms the conditions of His will. There was only one "no-no" and yet Eve chose deliberately to go against what God had so definitely told her!

What started trouble in her life? What starts it in our lives? The devil started promising her something. He began telling her lies. He dropped the thought into her mind that if she ate of the tree of the knowledge of good and evil that God would be happy because she would be as smart as God and have His same knowledge. He convinced her to go against what God had specifically said!

If the devil had been honest and straightforward (which he can never be) he would have said something like this, "Eve, I'm the one God threw out of heaven. Join me so you will die, then we can really have a ball together!" The devil is always smarter than that, although he doesn't have a single new trick up his sleeve – he keeps on using the old ones.

The first thing that happened was that the devil put a little tiny thought in Eve's mind. That little thought grew as she dwelt on it, and then it became a tiny little desire to disobey God. It really wasn't a desire to disobey God – it probably was just a desire to see if the devil was right!

Her thoughts probably went something like this: "I wonder if that really was God? I wonder why God would have told me not to eat this when it looks like it's good? That probably wasn't God after all, it was probably just my imagination." The devil didn't mention evil. He merely told her that she and Adam would be as gods. It's natural to want the best things in life, so she probably thought this was the "best" in life.

God said one thing, the devil said another. It's the same today!

Eve finally gave in to the temptation and decided to eat the fruit. It was not just the eating of the fruit that separated her from God; it was the thought, the decision, "I WILL GO AHEAD AND EAT IT!"

She first decided in her heart, then confessed it with her mind and then she ate it. This outward expression of an inward thought in her mind removed her from the will of God and God's abundant life. God's prosperity was taken from her.

Did she know what God's will was?

Certainly! God had told her specifically, but she didn't listen to God. She didn't obey God.

Doing what God wants us to do is the WILL of God!

Doing what WE want to do is NOT the will of God!

When you're doing the will of God, all of God's promises become yours.

When you're obeying God, ALL of His promises become yours! ALL OF HIS BLESSINGS!

God will bless you with prosperity!

God will bless you with health!

God will bless you with an abundance of all things as long as you are in HIS will!

And here is the secret for staying in the will of God!

Get into the word of God! Find the verses that quicken your spirit and they will tell you exactly what to do. Then do it!

III John 11 said something specific to me when I was saved: *"Beloved, do not imitate what is evil, but what is good. He who does good is of God, but he who does evil has not seen God."*

I turned around and looked at sin and it made me sick. I turned away and ran as fast as I could in the other direction. Many people sit down as close to sin as they can once they get saved, but when I read that scripture, I ran as fast as I could in the opposite direction!

What is God's will? To do good and not do evil. That is God's will for your life. Simple, isn't it? In other words, God is telling you to get the sin out of your life and quit being evil. That is the will of God for you.

Many times people have come to us asking us to pray for them that God's will for their lives will be revealed, when their lives are so full of sin that there is no way God could tell them what He wants them to do. That verse is one of the easiest ways I know of to get your life lined up with God so that you can find out what He wants for you. *"Beloved, do not imitate what is evil, but what is good."* That means YOU! That means me!

I John 3:6,7 gives another tremendous bit of advice concerning the will of God: *"Whoever abides in Him does not sin. Whoever sins has neither seen Him nor known Him. Little children, let no one deceive you. He who practices righteousness is righteous, just as He is righteous."*

In other words, if we want to know the will of God, we've got to have fellowship with God, but we cannot have fellowship with Him and still walk in darkness. You have to walk in the light of God. But you might say, "I just don't have all the light that I need; I just don't know as much about the Bible as I should. God hasn't spoken to me very much."

What's the answer?

Get into the word of God. Get out of the darkness and walk in all the light you have at that particular moment when you are really seeking the will of God.

Many people say, "Well, does God want me to stay on the same job or does God want me to change or what does God want me to do? I feel He's calling me into the ministry!"

Get into the word of God and see what God has to say to you. *"Let each one remain in the same calling in which he was called"* (I Corinthians 7:20).

I was in the printing business when I was saved. I kept doing the same job I had always done, only better now that I was saved until, little by little, God began taking me away by providing speaking engagements. However, I stayed on until God – not Frances – took me out of the printing business!

Does it make any difference if I sin just a little bit?

When you know what the word of God says to you about holy living and you know what God has to say about obedience to Him, then you will know the answer to that question immediately! God does not want you to live according to the lusts of this world and the lusts of the flesh. God wants you to live according to what His word says, in a pure, holy, and also, a very exciting life!

"For this is the WILL OF GOD, that you should be consecrated – separated and set apart

for pure and holy living: that you should abstain and shrink from all sexual vice; That each one of you should know how to possess (control, manage) his own body (in purity, separated from things profane, and) in consecration and honor, Not (to be used) in the passion of lust, like the heathen who are ignorant of the true God and have no knowledge OF HIS WILL..." (I Thess. 4:3-5 Amp).

"But the firm foundation (laid by) God stands, sure and unshaken, bearing this seal (inscription): The Lord knows those who are His, and, Let every one who names (himself by) the name of the Lord give up all iniquity and stand aloof from it" (II Tim. 2:19 Amp).

Isn't God's will simple? He could have just said, "Quit sinning," and that would have been enough for us to know His will in regard to sin!

If you really want to know the will of God, take a look at what it says in the book of Revelation. *"Come out of her, my people, lest you share in her sins..."* (Rev. 18:4).

You will never be able to find the will of God as long as you are trying to live in the world and as long as you are trying to partake of the sin of the world.

Eve wanted to walk with God and she wanted to walk with the devil. She wanted to have the things God told her she could not have. She wanted God's blessings and the lure of the devil. You can't have both!

If you want to know the will of God, line up your life with the word of God and the word of God will line up with your life!

Here is some more good advice directly from the mouth of God: *"Do not gather and heap up and store for yourselves treasures on earth, where moth and rust and worm consume and destroy, and where thieves break through and steal; But gather and heap up and store for yourselves treasures in heaven, where neither moth nor rust nor worm consume and destroy, and where thieves do not break through and steal; For where your treasure is, there will your heart be also"* (Matt. 6:19-21 Amp).

Where does God say to put your money? In the gold and silver of this world, in the perishable things of this world? His word says to store up for yourselves treasures in heaven because that's where your heart is going to be. If you put your trust in the things of this world that's right where your heart is going to be, but God tells us specifically where to put our treasures! Glory! How simple can the Christian life be!

God's will is so beautifully expressed in Matthew 6:25-33 in the Living Bible: *"So My counsel is: Don't worry about things – food, drink, and clothes. For you already have life and a body – and they are far more important than what to eat and wear. Look at the birds! They don't worry about what to eat – they don't need to sow or reap or store up food – for your heavenly Father feeds them. And you are far more valuable to him than they are. Will all your worries add a single moment to your life?*

"And why worry about your clothes? Look at

the field lilies! They don't worry about theirs. Yet King Solomon in all his glory was not clothed as beautifully as they. And if God cares so wonderfully for flowers that are here today and gone tomorrow, won't he more surely care for you, O men of little faith? So don't worry at all about having enough food and clothing. Why be like the heathen? For they take pride in all these things and are deeply concerned about them. But your heavenly Father already knows perfectly well that you need them, and he will give them to you IF YOU GIVE HIM FIRST PLACE IN YOUR LIFE AND LIVE AS HE WANTS YOU TO."

Is God's will for you to worry?

No!

When God tells you not to worry, He adds a real gem to it by saying, *"Will all your worries add a single moment to your life?"*

Who does the worrying?

The heathen!

Is God's will for you to worry like the heathen? No, no, no!

If you want to be in the perfect will of God, STOP WORRYING!

The word says, *"But without faith it is impossible to please Him, for he who comes to God must believe that He is, and that He is a rewarder of those who diligently seek Him"* (Hebrews 11:6).

To be in the will of God, start believing that He is a rewarder of them that diligently seek Him! Start saying, "God is going to reward me. God is going to reward me. God is rewarding me because I am diligently seeking Him!"

You might even go so far as to say, "I'm prospering because God is a rewarder of them who diligently seek Him. I'm a seeker, so God is prospering me!" Start seeing yourself prosperous!

God's will is for you to *"prosper in all things and be in health, just as your souls prospers"* (III John 2).

Is God's will for you to be in poverty and full of sickness!

NO, NO, NO!!!

If you had a rich relative die and leave you as an heir, their wish or their "will" would be that you have whatever they have. They might leave you antiques, they might leave you musical instruments, they might leave you cash, but if that rich relative made you the heir to the estate, everything in it would belong to you!

God's will is all written down. He made His Last Will and Testament in the form of the Old and New Testaments, and with this will that God has put into writing for us, we have every single direction He has for us written down so we can refer to it at all times. We have "GOD'S WILL, probated by Jesus!"

When we obey the word of God and do what God says in His word, then that is the will of God.

"A new commandment I give to you, that you love one another; as I have loved you, that you also love one another" (John 13:34).

What is God's will?

That we fight and scratch, complain and gossip, criticize one another, hate each other and try to destroy each other?

NO, NO, NO!

God's perfect will is that we love one another!

"Heal the sick, cleanse the lepers, raise the dead, cast out demons. Freely you have received, freely give" (Matthew 10:8).

How long has it been since you laid hands on the sick and healed them? If you are not out doing that, then you're not fully in God's will.

How long has it been since you cast out devils? That's God's will for your life. If you're not out doing that, but running when the subject of casting out devils is mentioned, then you are not in the perfect will of God! Get busy!

"There is therefore now no condemnation to those who are in Christ Jesus, who do not walk according to the flesh, but according to the Spirit. For the law of the Spirit of life in Christ Jesus has made me free from the law of sin and death" (Romans 8:1,2).

What is God's will in this instance? For us to walk with our heads held high because there is no one to judge us guilty of wrong because we are in Christ Jesus! There is no condemnation in our lives whatsoever.

We have been set free from the law of sin and death! God's will is for us to rejoice because we have been totally and completely, once and for all, set free from the law of sin and death! Condemnation? Absolutely not! There is NO condemnation of any kind.

"But you don't know what I've done in the past!" Who cares? God has forgiven you and if God can forgive you, you ought to be able to forgive yourself.

What is God's will? To walk and live with no condemnation in our lives whatsoever. To walk after the Spirit!

Further down in Romans 8 is one of the greatest chapters in the Bible to let you know God's will! *"So then, brethren, we are debtors, but not to the flesh [we are not obligated to our carnal nature], to live [a life ruled by the standards set up by the dictates] of the flesh. For if you live according to [the dictates of] the flesh, you will surely die. But if through the power of the [Holy] Spirit you are [habitually] putting to death (making extinct, deadening) the [evil] deeds prompted by the body, you shall [really and genuinely] live forever* (Romans 8:12,13 Amp).

What is God's will? It is for us to remember that we are not obligated to that old carnal nature. We don't have to do the things the devil tells us to do. God's will is that we believe that. *"Greater is he that is in us than he that is in the world"* (I John 4:4).

God's will is for us to believe that *"we are more than conquerors through him that loved us"* (Romans 8:37).

God's will is for us to act like the conquerors that we really are!

God's will is for us to believe His word and to act like we believe it!

God doesn't want us running around, sniffling all over the place, crying and saying, "I just don't think God loves me. Nothing good ever happens to me. Look at poor little me!"

God wants us to stand on His promise, *"For I am persuaded that neither death, nor life, nor angels, nor principalities nor powers, nor things present nor things to come, nor height nor depth, nor any other created thing, shall be able to separate us from the love of God which is in Christ Jesus our Lord"* (Romans 8:38,39).

Nothing, nothing, NOTHING can ever separate us from the love of God!

What is God's will for our lives? To believe that there is absolutely nothing in the entire world that can separate us from Him – except our own unbelief!

"Christ has redeemed us from the curse of the law, having become a curse for us (for it is written, 'Cursed is everyone who hangs on a tree') that the blessing of Abraham might come upon the Gentiles in Christ Jesus..." (Gal. 3:13,14).

What is God's will for our lives? To accept the fact that we have been redeemed from the curse of the law. What is the curse of the law? Sickness, poverty and separation from God!

What are the blessings of Abraham that belong to us because we have been redeemed from the curse of the law?

Health, prosperity and eternal life! That's God's will for our lives!

We've been redeemed!

We've been set free!

All the promises God made to Abraham belong to you and me. That's God's will for your life and mine!

Did you ever get to the place where you felt absolutely nothing was working right in your life? Did you ever have a sickness where you didn't seem to be able to manifest the healing that you knew was yours?

Did you ever have a financial problem that you felt was insurmountable?

God gave me revelation knowledge about a scripture which I had never seen before in that particular light. If you have any problem in your life which seems to be a mountain too big to cast to one side, this is just for you:

"Why is my pain perpetual, and my wound incurable, refusing to be healed?" That could mean your financial pain, physical pain, marital pain, your offspring pains, job pain or any situation in your life which is not right. *"Will you indeed be to me as a deceitful brook, like waters that fail and are uncertain? Therefore thus says the Lord (to Jeremiah)..."* but to me he said (to Frances) *"...If you return (give up this mistaken tone of distrust and despair), then I will give you again a settled place of quiet and safety, and you shall be My minister; and if you separate the precious from the vile..."* now God, what in my life could be vile? I can't think of anything that You would consider vile! What is it, God?

Be careful when you say that, because look at His answer: *"(cleansing your own heart from unworthy suspicions concerning God's faithful-*

ness), you shall be as My mouthpiece" (Jeremiah 15:19 Amp). Have you ever been suspicious concerning God's faithfulness? God really underscored that to me!

God's will is for you to get all of those unworthy suspicions concerning His faithfulness out of your mind, your heart, your body and your soul. We let doubt and despair creep into our lives, and before we know it we have in our hearts what God calls "vileness."

God's will is for you to trust Him in all things, and at all times, and to stop the devil from making those inroads into your life through unbelief!

Here's another gem if you've ever been persecuted for what you believe!

"Blessed – happy, to be envied, and spiritually prosperous (that is, with life-joy and satisfaction in God's favor and salvation, regardless of your outward conditions) – are you when people revile you and persecute you and say all kinds of evil things against you falsely on My account. Be glad and supremely joyful, for your reward in heaven is great (strong and intense), for in this same way people persecuted the prophets who were before you" (Matt. 5:11,12 Amp).

What is God's will for your life? You are to have life, joy and satisfaction in God's favor and salvation when people persecute you. When they talk against you for believing in the baptism with the Holy Spirit and speaking in tongues, God's will is for you to rejoice, and be not only a little joyful, but supremely joyful, which means to the highest extent.

I always thought when the beatitudes ended, they ended. I always wondered when I read the next verse what salt had to do with them. It always seemed that verse was a little out of context, but while we were flying far out over the Pacific on the way to Australia, God revealed that it all belonged together. Watch how it ties together for God's will for your life:

"You are the salt of the earth, but if salt has lost its taste – its strength, its quality – how can its saltness be restored? It is not good for anything any longer but to be thrown out and trodden underfoot by men" (Matt. 5:13 Amp).

God said that if you don't believe what you say when men persecute you and become a people pleaser and let them talk you into shutting up, then you are no longer the salt of the earth. You will be absolutely no good for his kingdom, but you'll be thrown out to be trodden under the feet of the men who have persecuted you!

I was so excited I could have almost jumped out of the plane 37,000 feet in the air – but I didn't. Instead I began to pound on Charles to share with him what God had revealed to me, then I continued reading, *"You are the light of the world. A city set on a hill cannot be hid"* (Matt. 5:14 Amp).

God wants us to let our lights shine in a world of darkness. He doesn't want us to be intimidated by the devil's disciples. If we're going to be salt in the kingdom of God, we've got to be salt. We've got to let our lights shine because we are the light of the world!

Get out that polishing cloth and shine up that light of yours because God's will is for you to let yourself be a beacon light. Turn that voltage up and let your light shine brighter than ever before!

When we arrived in Australia, we shared this bit of revelation knowledge with our friends and the first thing that was said was, "When does salt do the most seasoning?" He answered, "Salt penetrates in cooking or heat." Faith grows when you're under fire or "the heat's on!" Hallelujah!

"But I tell you, Love your enemies and pray for those who persecute you" (Matt. 5:44 Amp). Glory to God, what is His will for your life? To love those enemies and pray for those who persecute you! Get busy right now and see what happens to you when you do! You'll really discover God's will in a hurry when you start loving your enemies and praying for those who persecute you!

We were severely persecuted when we wrote God's beautiful messages in the book ANGELS ON ASSIGNMENT. But because God had confirmed to us by many signs and wonders and even angel visitations – and by His word – we had continual life, joy in knowing this was God's will, and we prayed for those who persecuted us.

"Those who let themselves be controlled by their lower nature live only to please themselves, but those who follow after the Holy Spirit find themselves doing those things that please God. Following after the Holy Spirit leads to life and peace, but following after the old nature leads

to death, because the old sinful nature within us is against God. It never did obey God's laws and it never will. That's why those who are still under the control of their old sinful selves, bent on following their old evil desires, can never please God" (Rom. 8:5-8 TLB).

What is God's will in this instance? That you follow after the Holy Spirit. Why? Because if you decide to please self what's going to happen? Exactly what God's Word says – you're going to be miserable. Is that God's will for you? No, No, No!

The Holy Spirit is reading God's will and testament to you! He will tell you where to go and what to do. Your old nature, your desires, your "self," wants to pull away from the will of God, for we "naturally love to do evil things that are just the opposite of things that the Holy Spirit tells us to do!" Our old nature constantly says, "A cigarette won't hurt you - a social drink is all right!"

The Holy Spirit says, *"I beseech you therefore, brethren, by the mercies of God, that you present your bodies a living sacrifice, holy, acceptable to God, which is your reasonable service"* (Romans 12:1).

How holy and acceptable are you to God when you reek and stink like cigarettes, or when you've got alcohol oozing out of all your pores? Are you holy and acceptable to God when your display of "Christ in You" is distorted by an unforgiving or nasty attitude?

What is God's will for us? That we present our bodies acceptable to God. How plain and simple can the will of God be?

The Holy Spirit says, *"And do not be conformed to this world, but be transformed by the renewing of your mind, that you may prove what is that good and acceptable and perfect will of God"* (Romans 12:2).

What is God's will for us? That we don't follow after the things of this world – that we don't have to go along with all the external, superficial customs which this world says are the "in" things but that we begin to put our minds on the higher things of God and that we begin to change our ideals and that we change our attitudes about the real values in life.

The will of God, generally speaking, is the exact opposite of the old nature, yet the Bible says to take delight in the Lord and He will give you the desires of your heart (Psalm 37:4).

If you're following after the Holy Spirit, and you want to please God, then God, through His word and by His Spirit, is going to put the desires in your heart. You will understand from the Bible what pleases God, what makes Him happy and suddenly that desire He puts in your heart to make Him happy will come forth, and you will speak it out – you'll say it, you'll do it – you'll follow after the Holy Spirit and you'll have the very desires of your own heart because God put them there through His word!

Before I was saved, the desires of my heart were to go boating, fishing and playing golf on Sundays. I always had the best excuses in the world for not going to church on Sundays. One of my favorites was: "I can be just as good a Christian out on the golf course as I can be in church." Or maybe I'd say, "I can worship God just as much out on the ocean as I can in church!" Just anything to get out of going to church!

You CAN worship God just as much on a golf course – but you won't!

You CAN worship God just as much out on a boat – but you won't!

Because the will of God is that you assemble yourselves with other Christians. Today, Charles and I would like to spend every day in church, and we spend the majority of all of our days in church services! As I finish this book, I'm anticipating the next two weeks where we'll be having one, two or three services each day. We can hardly wait to pack our suitcases and get going because the desire of our hearts is to follow after the Holy Spirit. Who placed those desires in our hearts? God did, because He said if we take delight in Him, He Himself would give us, or plant within our very own hearts, the desires He wants us to have, and then give them to us by fulfilling them! Glory!

There are five basic ingredients in being in the will of God at all times. In the third chapter of John, Jesus said, "You must be born again." The will of God is that you be born again; that your spirit be made alive in Christ Jesus by accepting and believing on the name of the Lord Jesus. When you have done that, that is step number one in the will of God. It is not the will of God that you just sit down after you are born again, but that's the start.

The second thing that causes you to be in the will of God and to stay in the will of God, is to meditate in the word of God.

When I was saved, God put a hunger in my heart for the word of God which has never been satisfied. I don't care how many times I read and reread the Bible, I find new and exciting things in it all the time. I owned a printing company when I was saved and I sat beside a printing press many nights until five o'clock in the morning, just reading the word of God!

If you're in the will of God, you're going to be in the word of God – and if you're in the word of God, you're going to be in the will of God! That's a complicated thought, but read it over two or three times until you get the total meaning of it!

"For with the heart one believes to righteousness, and with the mouth confession is made to salvation" (Romans 10:10).

What is God's will for your life?

That you confess your salvation with your mouth! That you share the Good News with your own mouth which confirms your salvation! God's will is for you to be a real blabbermouth Christian, and not a secret service one! Start talking about what Jesus has done in your life and watch the blessings really begin to flow!

"And these signs will follow those who believe;… they will speak with new tongues" (Mark 16:17). That's the baptism with the Holy Spirit. That's God's will for your life, for you to have

power. He didn't let Jesus die for us to exist powerlessly in a world where we need all the power we can muster to resist the devil! That's God's will for you – to speak with new tongues! Lift your hands and begin to praise him, but not in a language you understand, and see what happens!

That's God's will – that brand new tongue with which to praise Him. Hallelujah! Glory to God!

The fifth thing we need to do is to make a total and complete commitment of our lives. I remember the day I got saved, I made a profound statement, "God, if you want what's left of this mess, you take me, but take ALL of me because I don't want a single bit of myself left!"

Sometimes we do these things in a different order than I have listed them, but that really doesn't make any difference – we just need to do ALL of them to be in the perfect will of God!

Wherever I open the Bible, I find more of God's instructions and his will: *"Rejoice always"* (I Thes. 5:16). That's God's perfect will for your life. And if the word says to rejoice evermore, that's exactly what I'm going to do! I'm going to be happy that I'm saved, I'm going to be glad-hearted continually, and I'm going to rejoice at all times, through all circumstances and under all conditions, because this is the will of God!

He says to *"Pray without ceasing"* (I Thes. 5:17), so I'm going to talk to God at all times because then I know I'm in His perfect will! I'm going to talk to Him when I'm driving down the highway, I'm going to "think" to Him when

I'm working, I'm going to meditate in His word, which is listening to Him, so I'm going to continually have Him on my mind instead of the things of the world!

I'm going to thank God in everything because I'm not going to look at things through natural eyes. I'm going to look at things through my spirit eyes and see them as God sees them. I'm not going to look at the mountains in my life. I'm going to look at the Mover because that is God's will for my life and yours!

One of the most exciting things in the will of God, is to fulfill what His Word says is yours. John 17:13 in the Living Bible says, *"now I am coming to you. I have told them* (my Bible says "Charles and Frances") *many things while I was with them so that they would be filled with my JOY."*

If Jesus said that I am filled with His joy, then I'm going to be filled with His joy. When I was a little girl going to the deadest church in the world, I used to stand there and peek up at the miserable looking "Christians" and I would think to myself, "I don't want to go to heaven because if that's what's in heaven, I couldn't stand to be with those crabs all the time!"

The people in the church were so miserable looking, I couldn't imagine any punishment much worse than having to spend all of eternity with them, so I made a great statement, "I want to go to hell so I'll be with all my friends!"

What an ambition – and all because not one single person ever told me about the joy of the

Lord!

What is God's will for your life?

To show the JOY of the Lord to those around you who may have never seen the real joy of the Christian life.

It's fun to be saved!

It's God's will to be saved!

It's God's will to enjoy your salvation!

It's God's will for you to pass that joy on to others!

It's God's will for you to prosper!

It's God's will for you to be in health!

It's God's will for you to have the abundant life!

It's God's will for you to be an overcomer!

It's God's will for you to have power over the devil!

It's God's will for you to speak in tongues!

It's God's will for you to be holy!

For the latest salvation reports in the World Evangelistic Census, or total video home churches, call: (713) 358-7575 or fax (281) 358-4130

E-mail: wec@cfhunter.org

Website: www.cfhunter.org